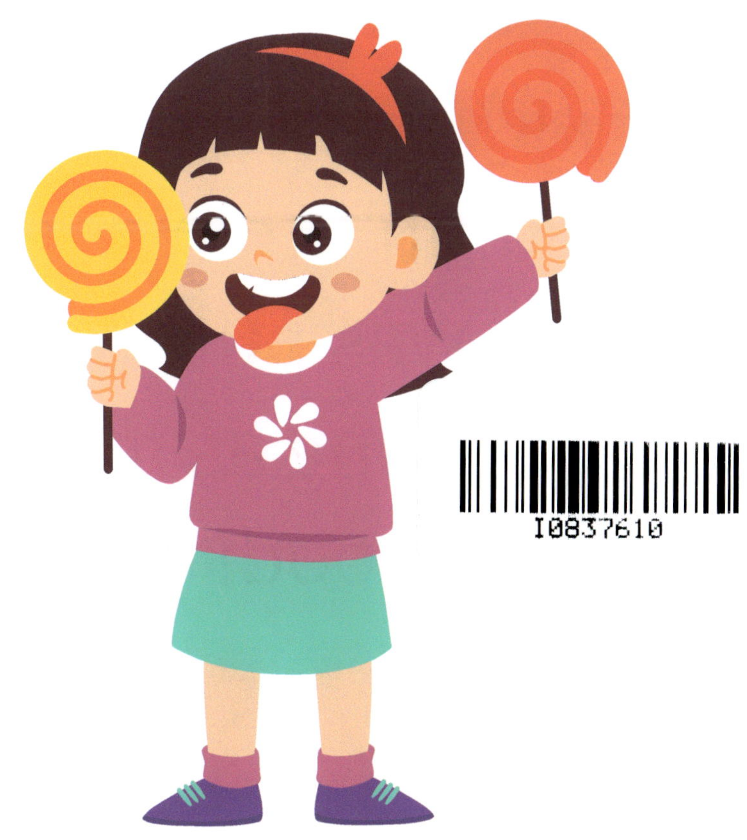

Once upon a time, in a land not too far away, there was a little girl named Charlie. Charlie loved to eat junk food and candy all day long.

She didn't think about what she was putting in her body, as long as it tasted good!

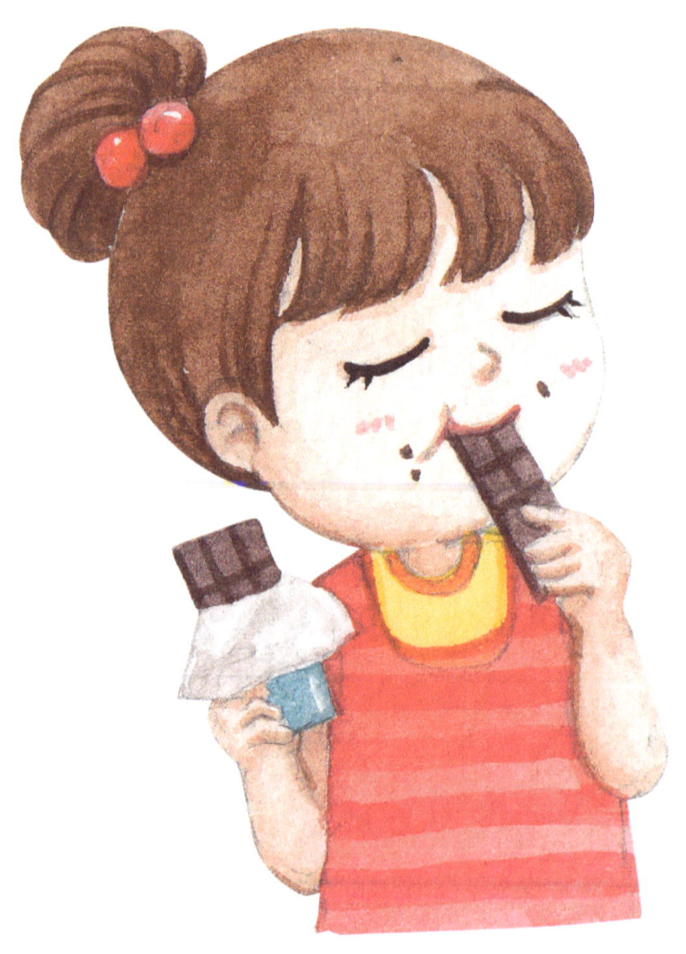

One day, while playing outside, Charlie started to feel tired and sluggish.

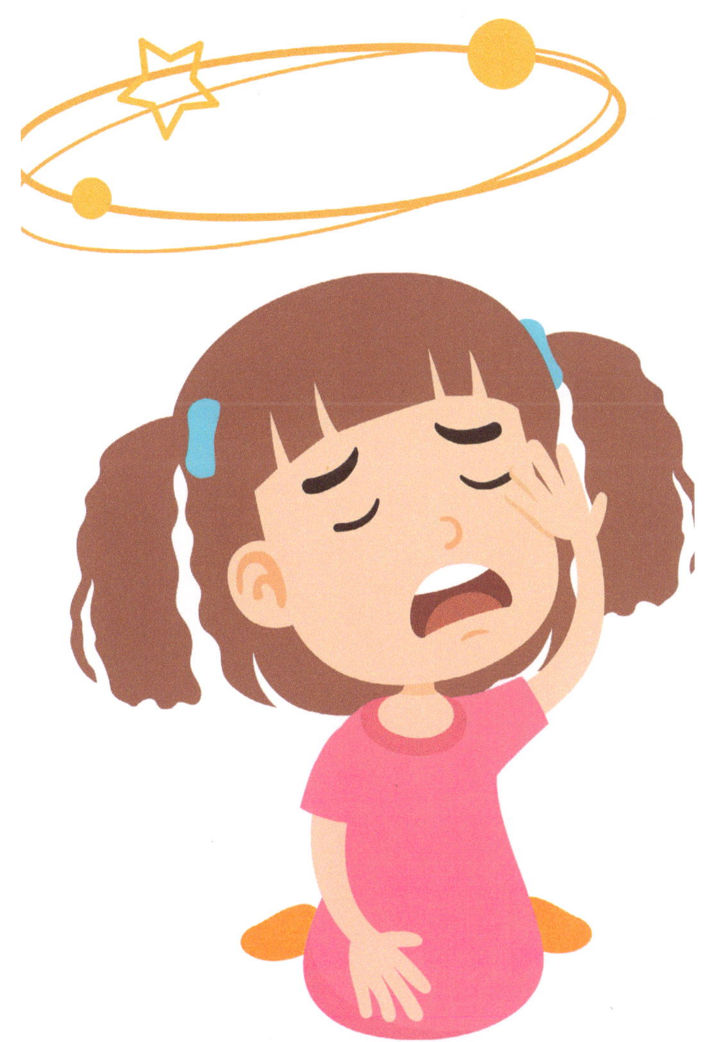

She couldn't run as fast as she used to, and her friends were starting to outpace her. She realized that maybe all the junk food wasn't making her feel so great after all.

Charlie decided to make a change and start eating healthy.

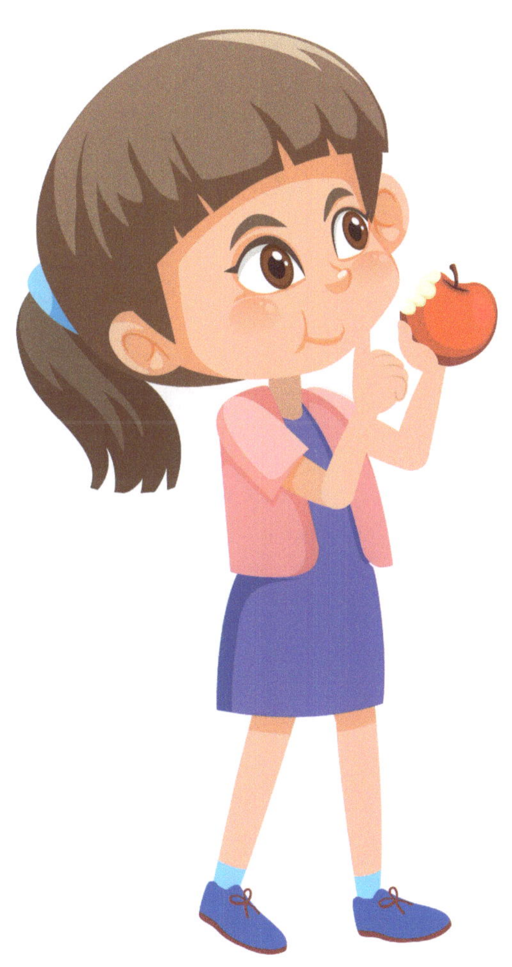

She asked her mom to take her to the grocery store, where they picked out lots of fruits, vegetables, and whole grains.

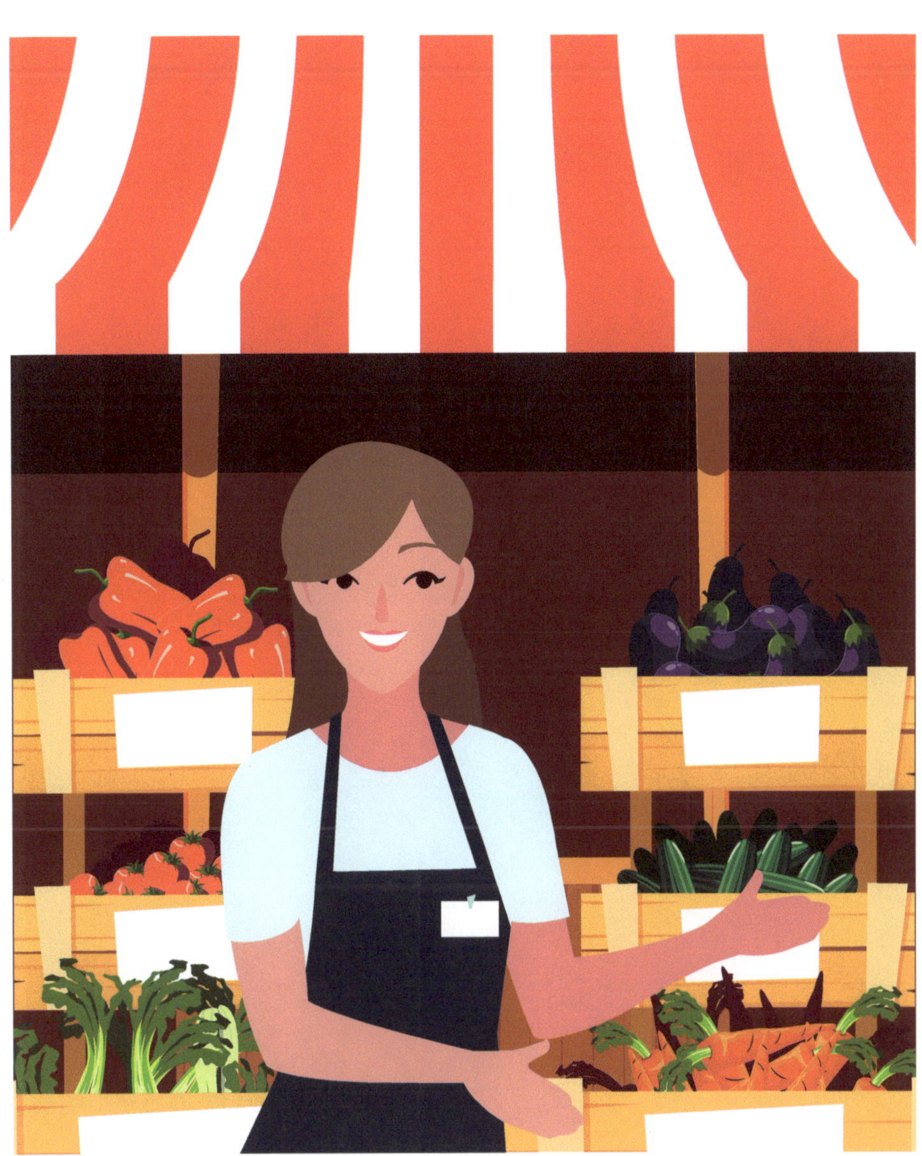

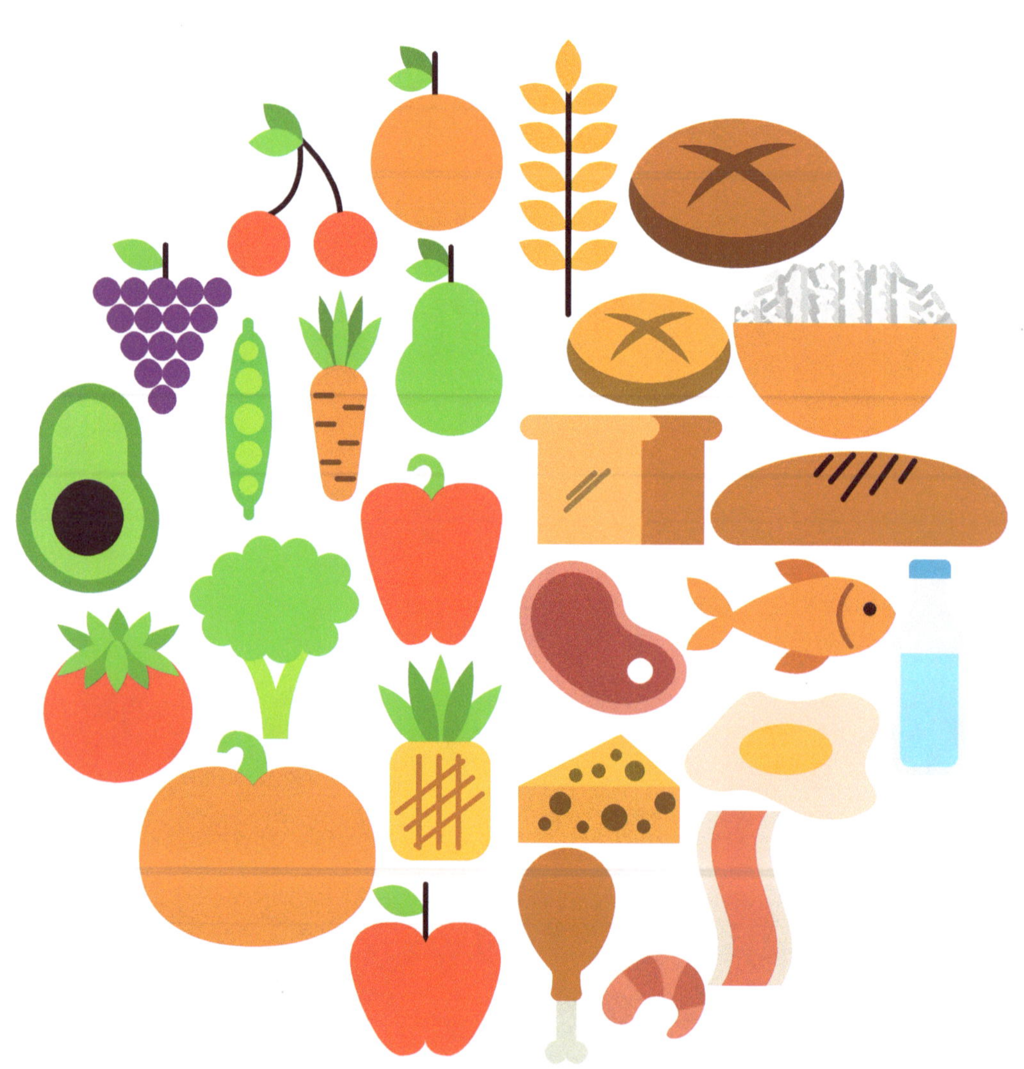

They also picked up some lean protein, like chicken and fish.

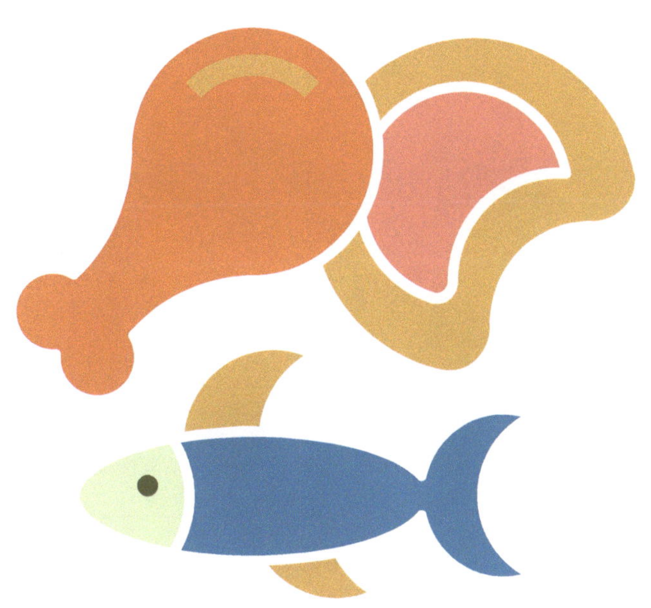

At first, Charlie wasn't sure about these new foods. She had never tasted things like kale or quinoa before!

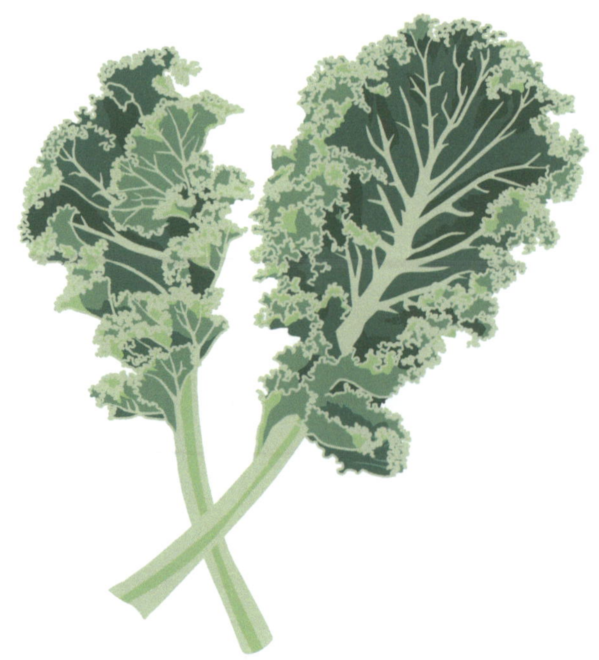

But she decided to give them a try, and to her surprise, she really liked them.

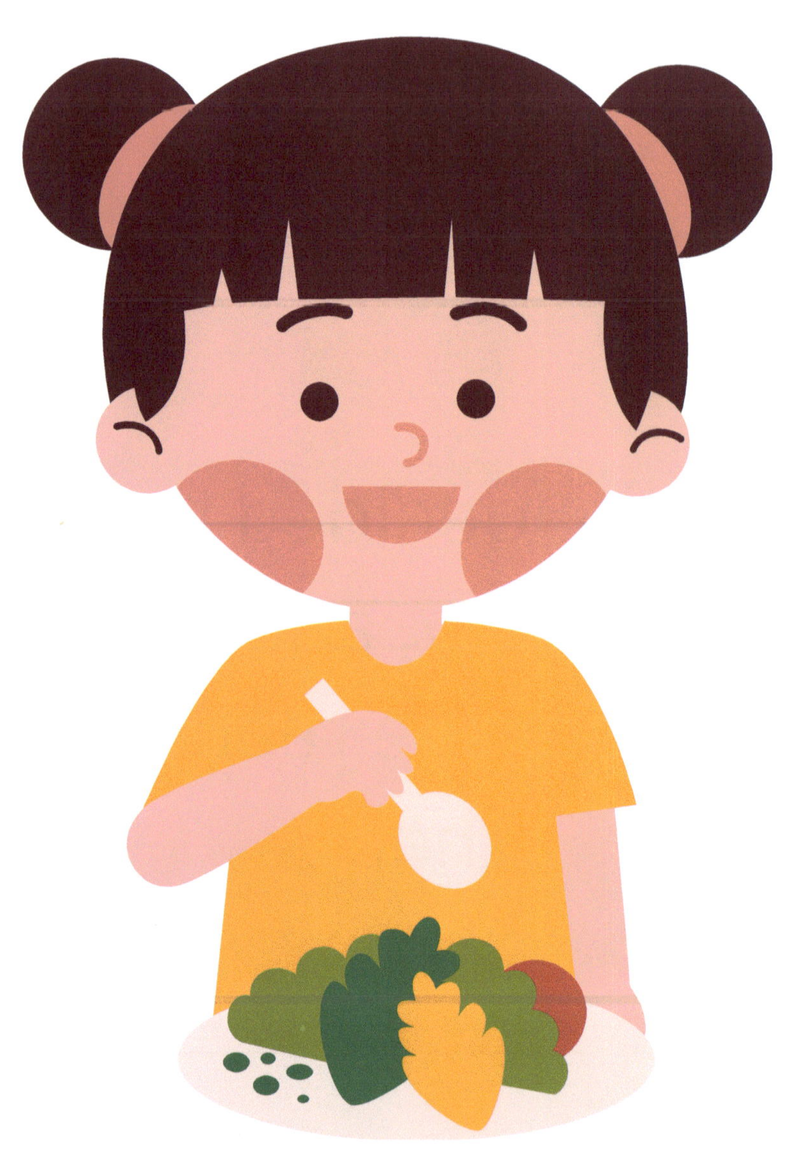

She felt better and more energized than ever before.

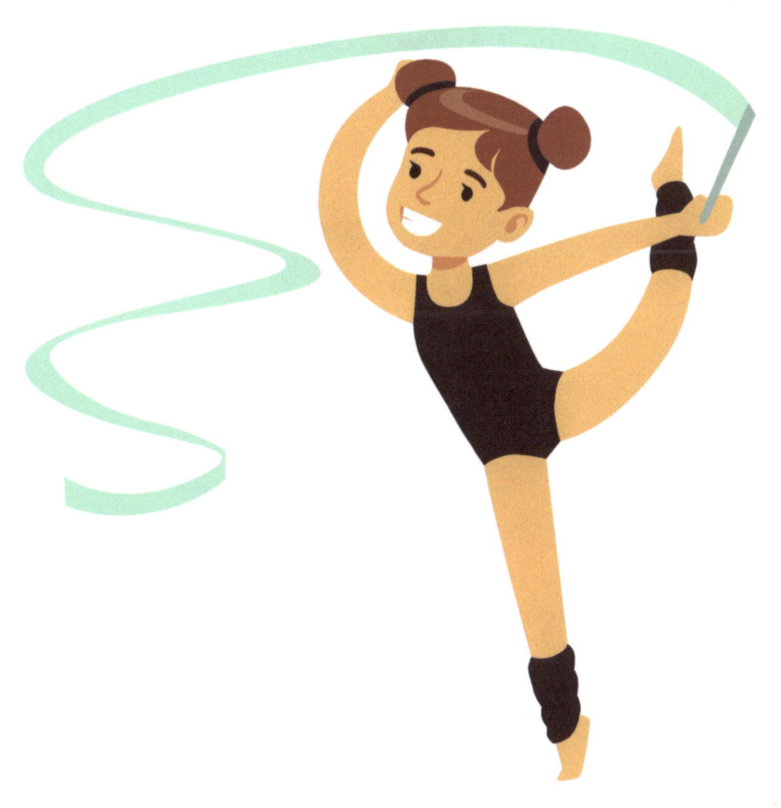

As the weeks went by, Charlie noticed that she was able to run faster and play longer with her friends.

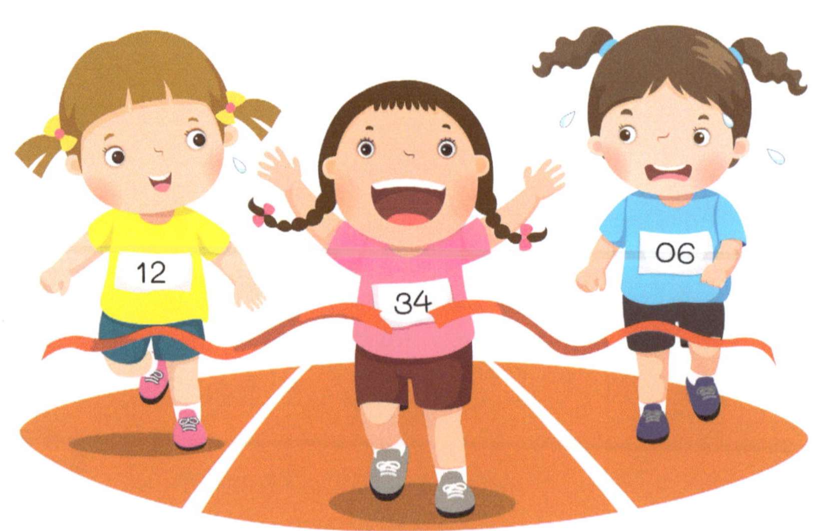

she was able to concentrate better in school, too.

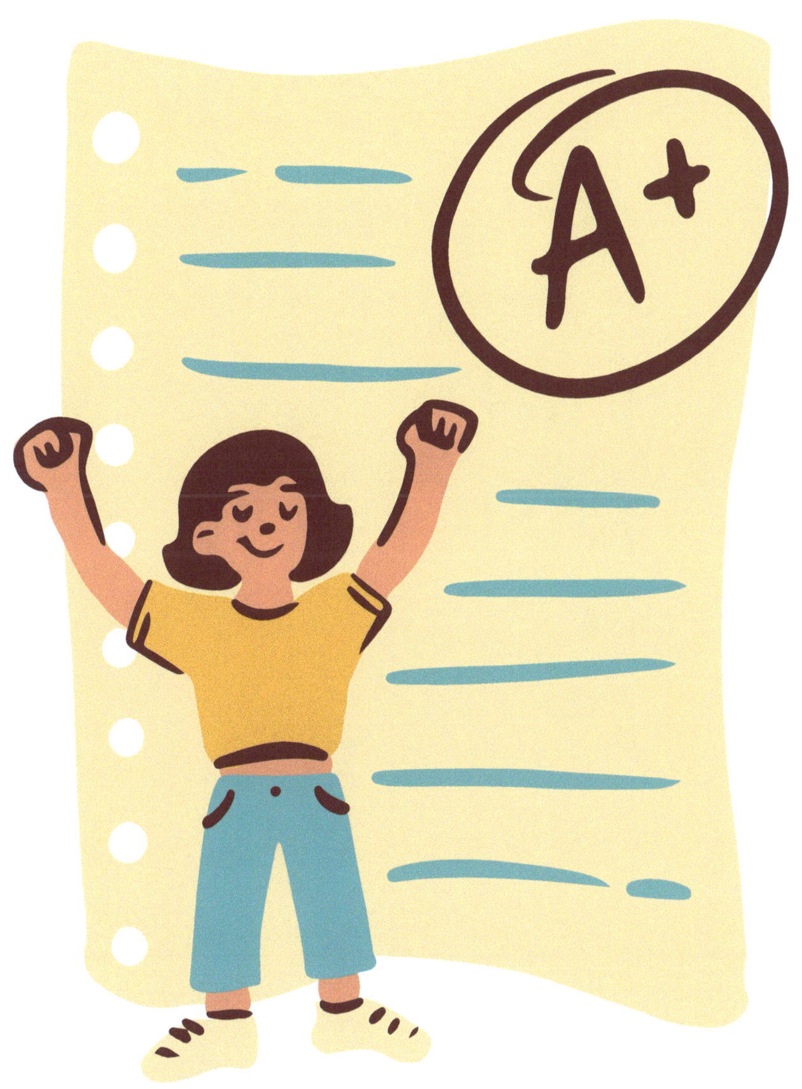

Her mom was happy to see her eating healthy, and even started cooking more healthy meals for the whole family.

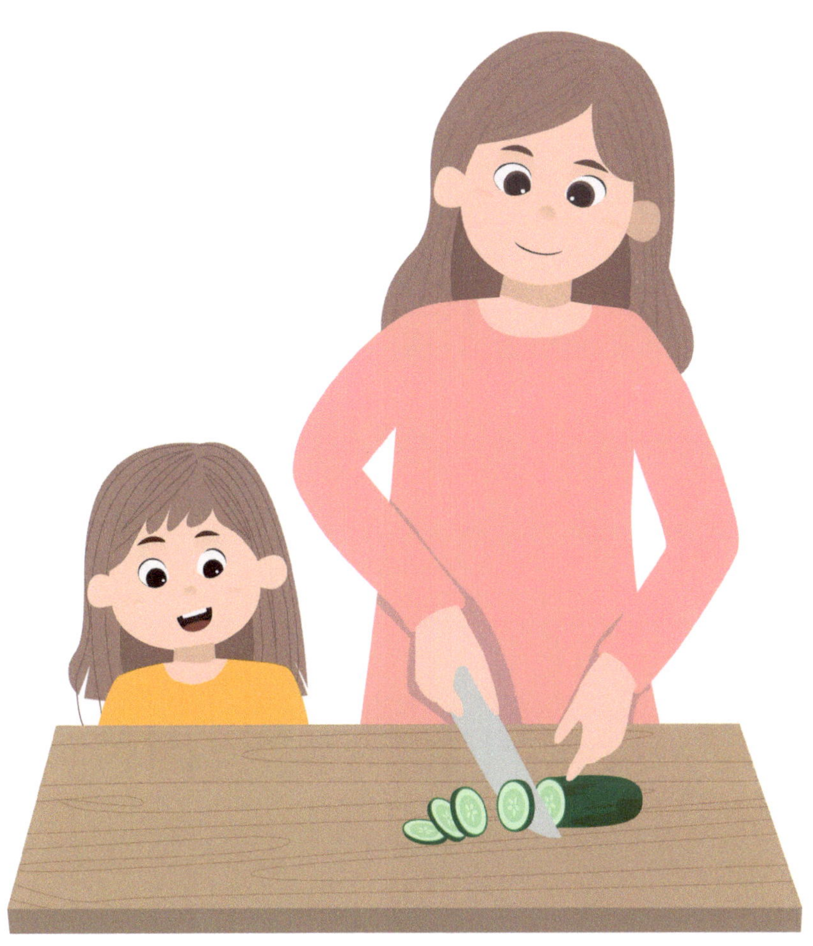

Charlie realized that eating healthy wasn't just good for her body, but it also made her feel happy and proud of herself.

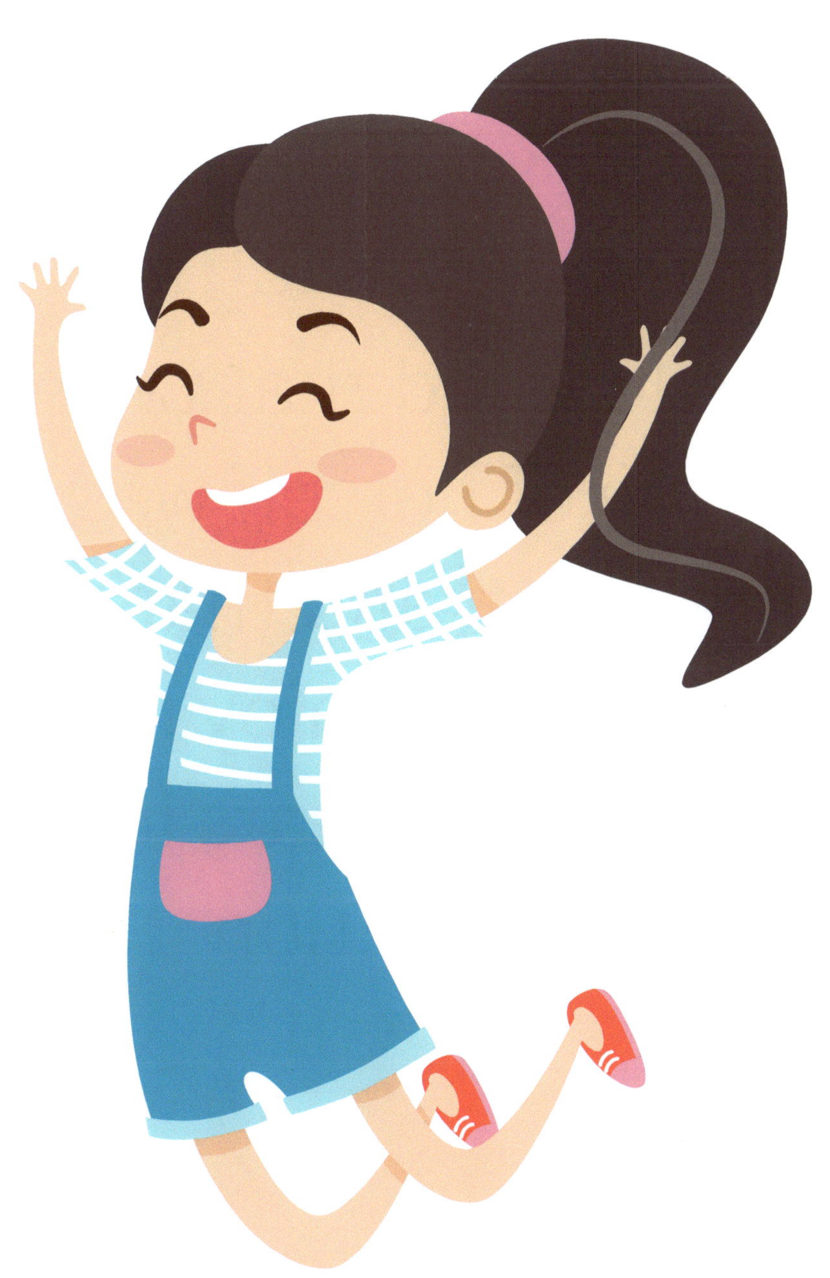

She learned that taking care of herself was important, and that she could still enjoy her favorite treats in moderation.

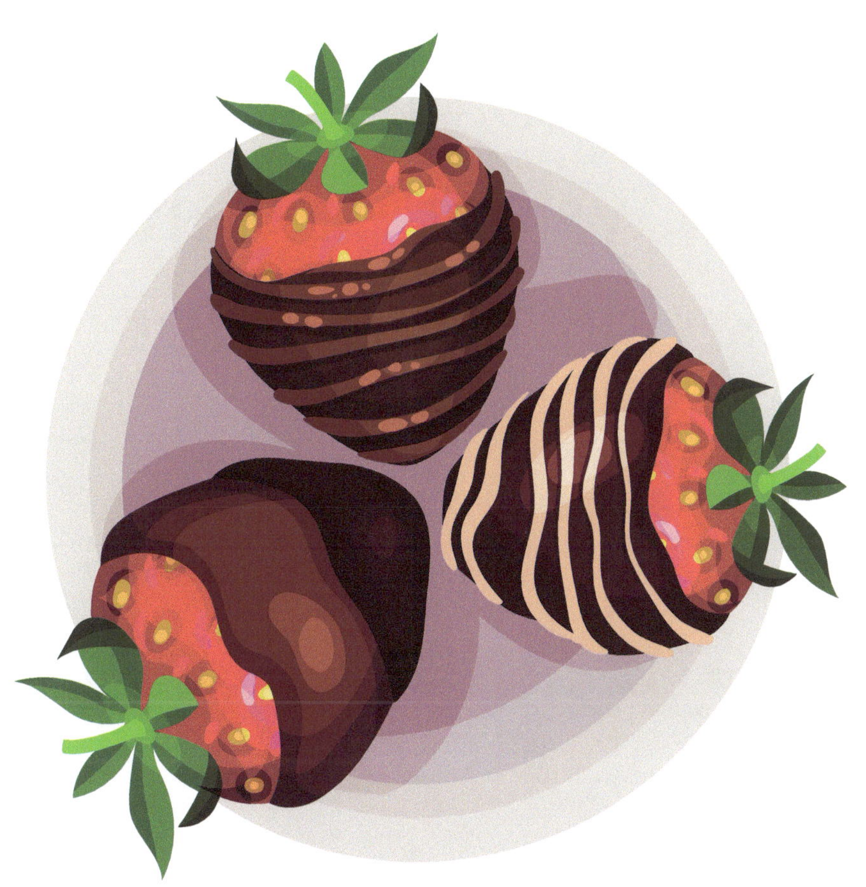

From that day on, Charlie made a promise to herself to always eat healthy and take care of her body.

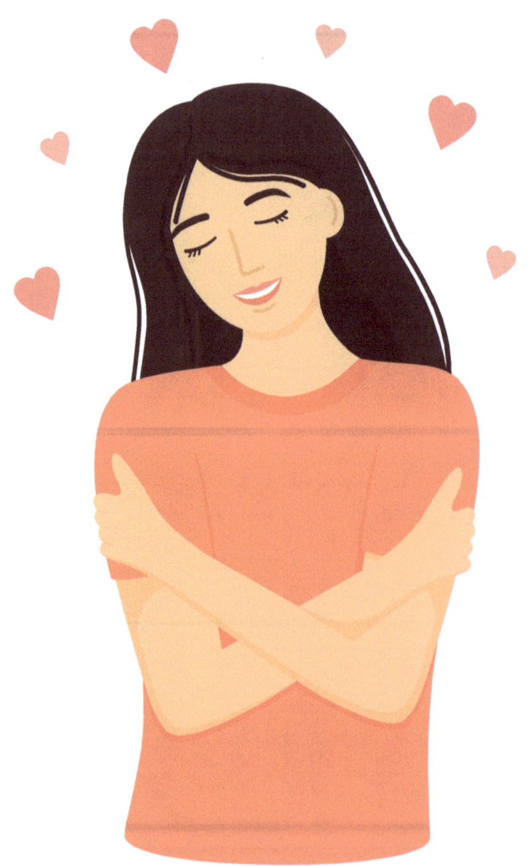

She knew that it was the key to living a happy and healthy life.

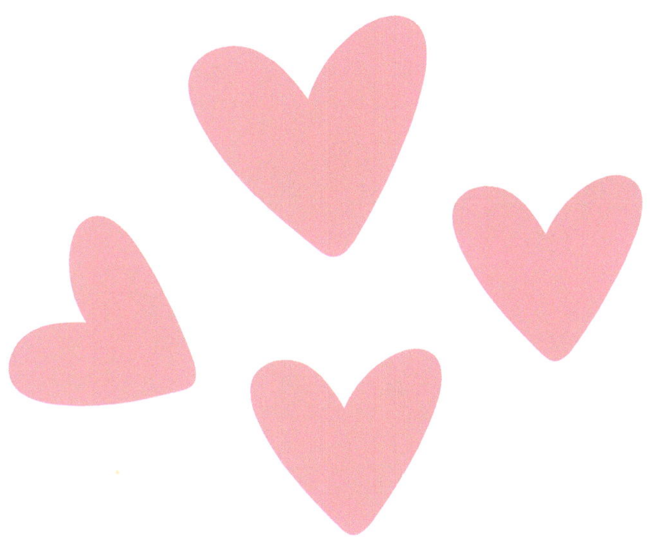

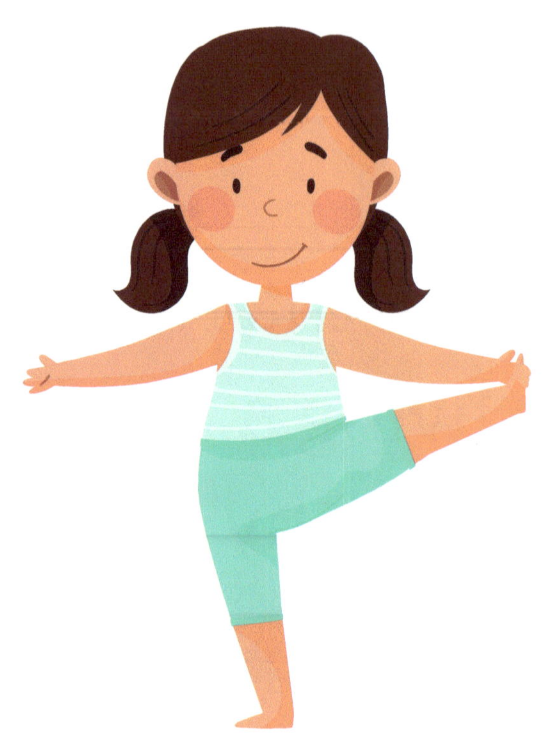
Be
HEALTHY
eat
HEALTHY

www.ingramcontent.com/pod-product-compliance
Lightning Source LLC
Chambersburg PA
CBHW040321240726
48664CB00006B/1589